INTRODUCTION

We all want that picture-perfect, glowing skin, but sometimes skin issues can stand in the way. No need to fret! Our ultimate guide has got you covered. We're diving deep into the most common skin problems, their triggers and the top-notch remedies to get your skin feeling happy and healthy. We're even helping you to build your own skincare routine! From acne to eczema, we've got the lowdown on how to give your skin the love it deserves.

Sophia

SOPHIA BOWES
SKINCARE ENTHUSIAST/ ENTREPRENEUR

LET'S DO IT!

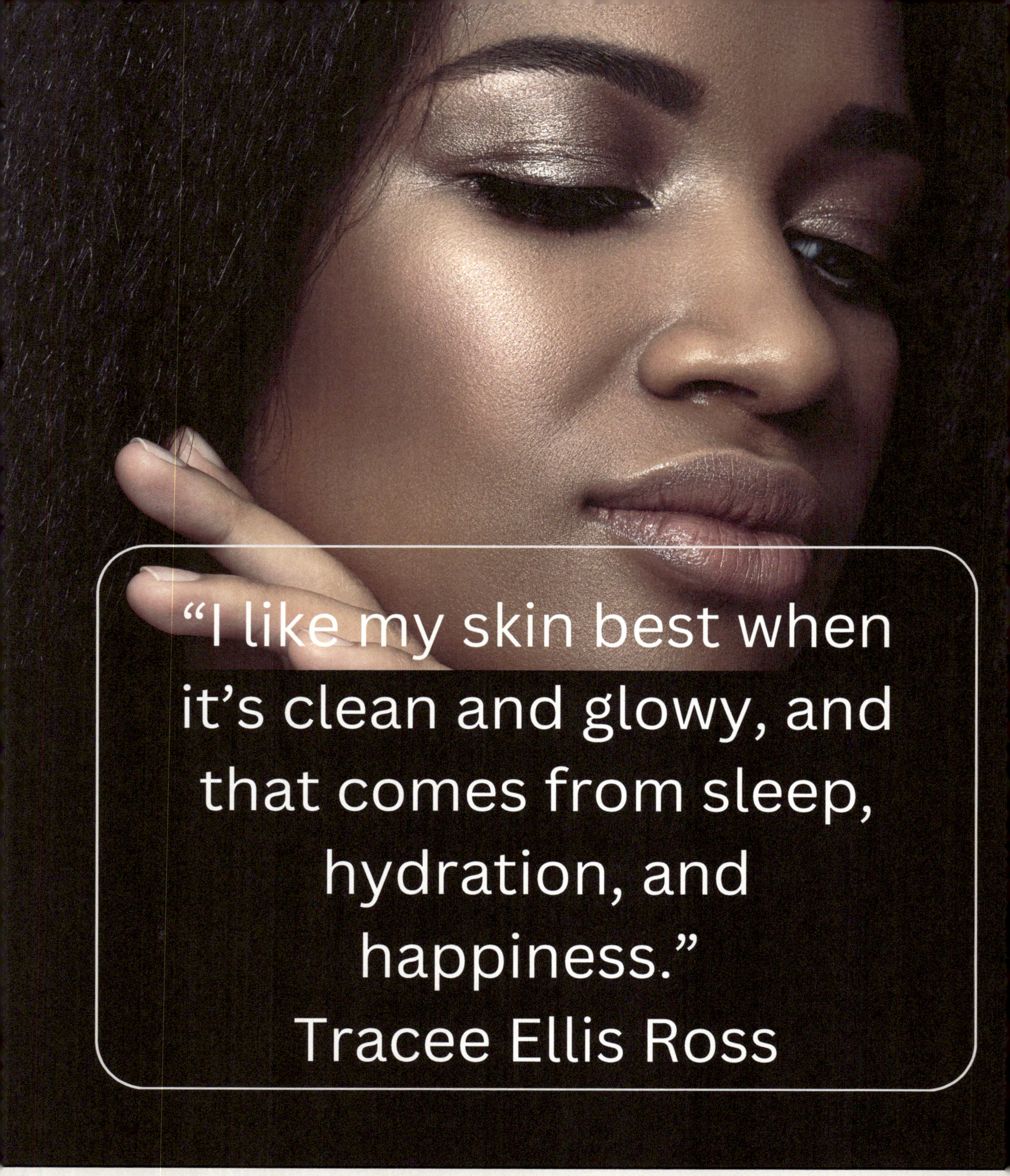

"I like my skin best when it's clean and glowy, and that comes from sleep, hydration, and happiness."
Tracee Ellis Ross

Table of 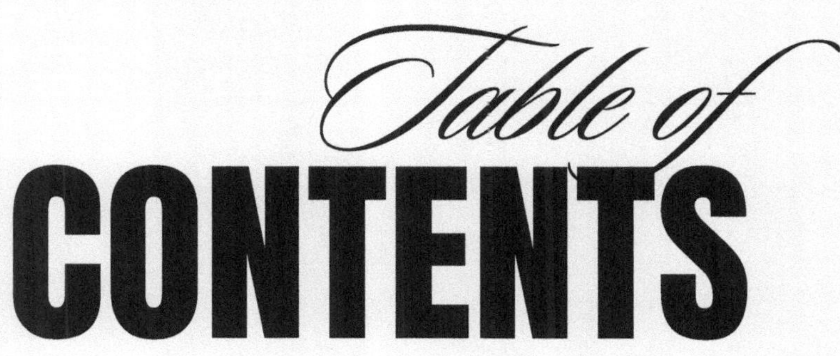
CONTENTS

01

UNDERSTANDING YOUR SKIN

Step right into the thrilling universe of skincare! This sweet chapter is all about the nitty-gritty of your beautiful skin.

02

COMMON SKIN ISSUES

Join us on a skin-tastic journey as we explore the most frequent skin concerns of all time!

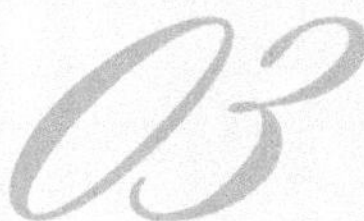

03

CAUSES OF SKIN ISSUES

Get ready to plunge into the deep end of the pool and explore a whole array of factors that could play a role in developing skin concerns.

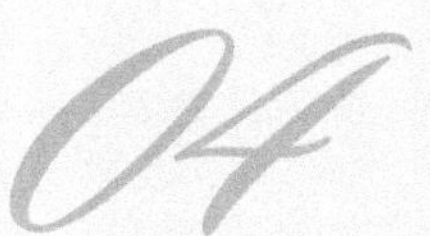

04

EFFECTIVE SOLUTIONS FOR RADIANT SKIN

This chapter will provide you with helpful tips and recommended products that can assist you in achieving radiant skin.

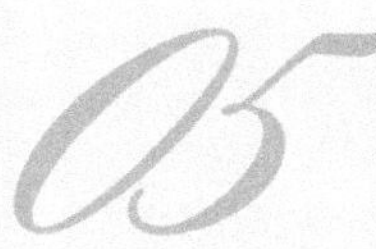

05

SKINCARE INGREDIENTS TO LOOK FOR

Welcome to the next chapter, where we'll spill the beans on how a handful of powerful ingredients can help you achieve that coveted glow-up!

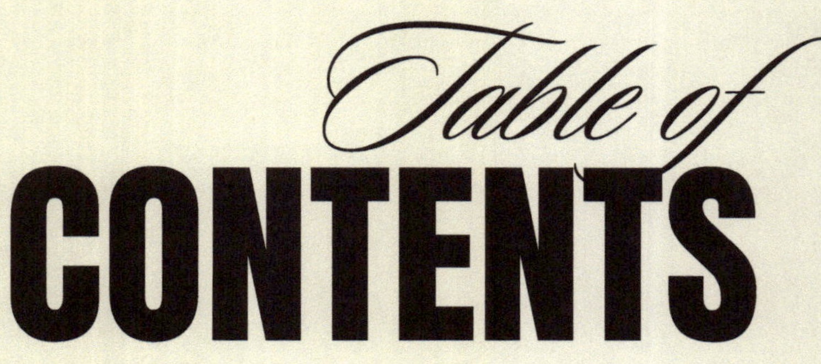

Table of CONTENTS

CHAPTER

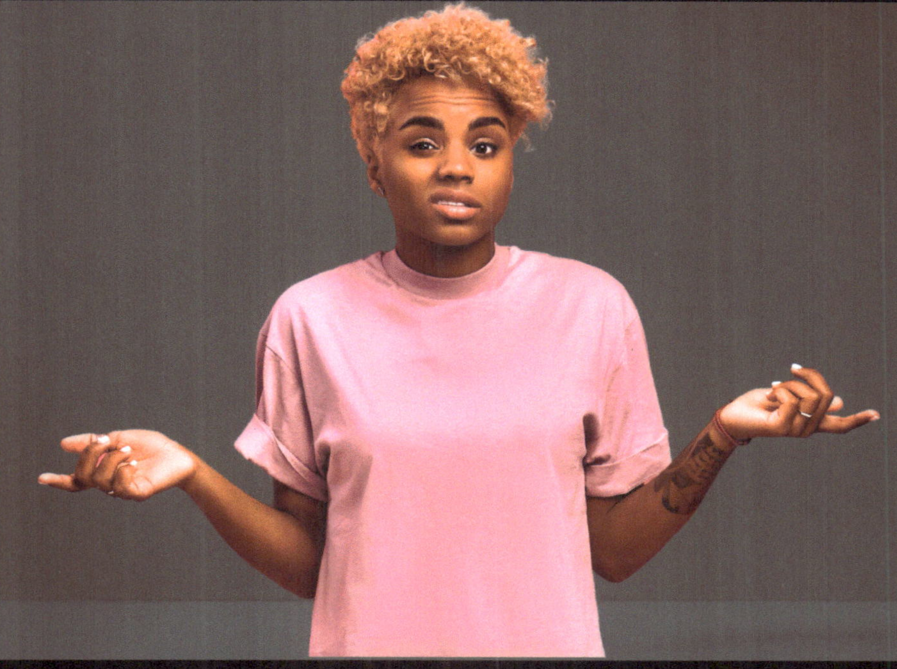

1

UNDERSTANDING YOUR SKIN | 1 PAGE

LET'S DO IT

UNDERSTANDING YOUR SKIN

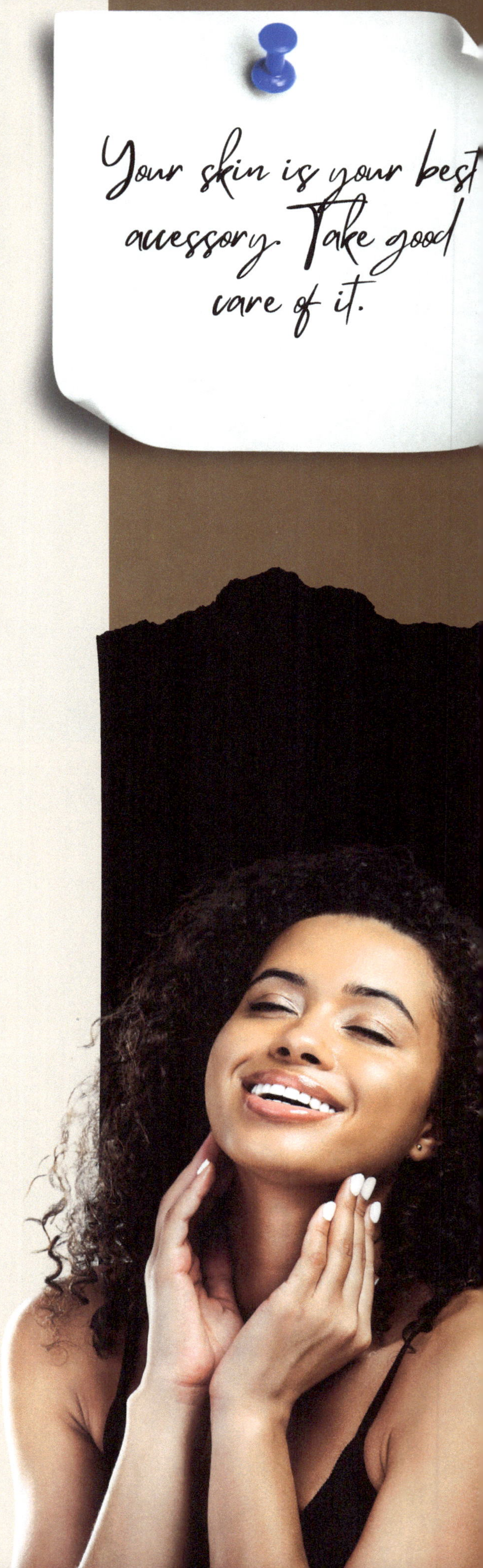

Before diving into specific skin problems and solutions, it's essential to understand the basics of your skin's structure, function, and different skin types.

Skin Structure

The skin is the largest organ of the body and consists of three main layers: the epidermis, dermis, and subcutis. The epidermis is the outermost layer, followed by the dermis, and the subcutis is the innermost layer.

Skin Function

The skin serves multiple functions, including protection from external elements, regulation of body temperature, sensation, and synthesis of vitamin D.

Skin Types

There are four primary skin types: normal, dry, oily, and combination. Each skin type has specific characteristics and requires tailored skincare routines and products.

Take our skin type quiz to learn your skin type <u>here</u> and write it down on the next page for future reference.

MY SKIN TYPE

CHAPTER

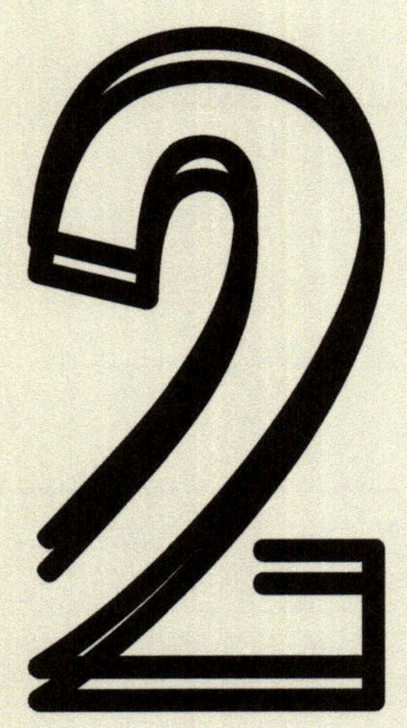

COMMON SKIN PROBLEMS

3 PAGES

LET'S DO IT

COMMON SKIN PROBLEMS

In this section, we will explore common skin problems that can affect anyone, regardless of their skin type or age. Understanding these skin problems will help you identify and address your specific concerns effectively.

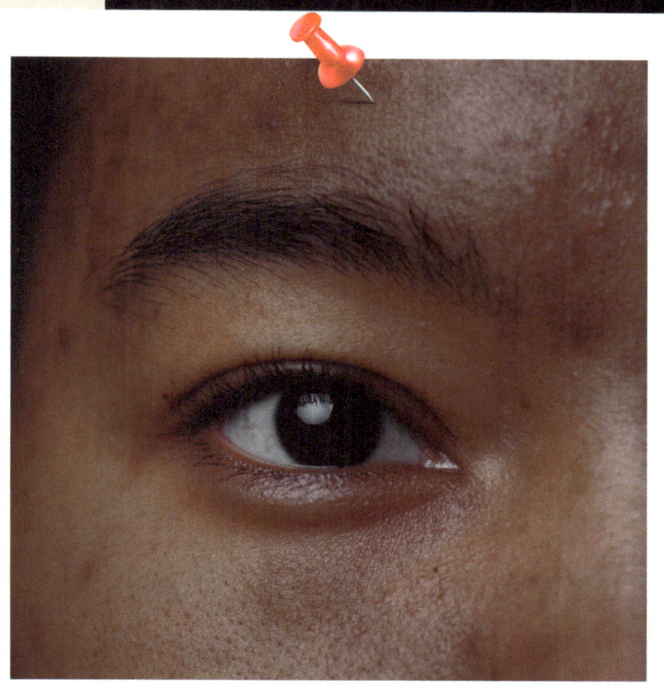

Acne

Acne is a prevalent skin condition characterized by the formation of pimples, blackheads, whiteheads, and cysts. It is commonly caused by excess oil production, clogged pores, bacteria, and inflammation.

Eczema

Eczema, also known as atopic dermatitis, is a chronic inflammatory skin condition. It is characterized by dry, itchy, and red patches on the skin. Eczema can be triggered by various factors, including genetics, allergies, and environmental factors.

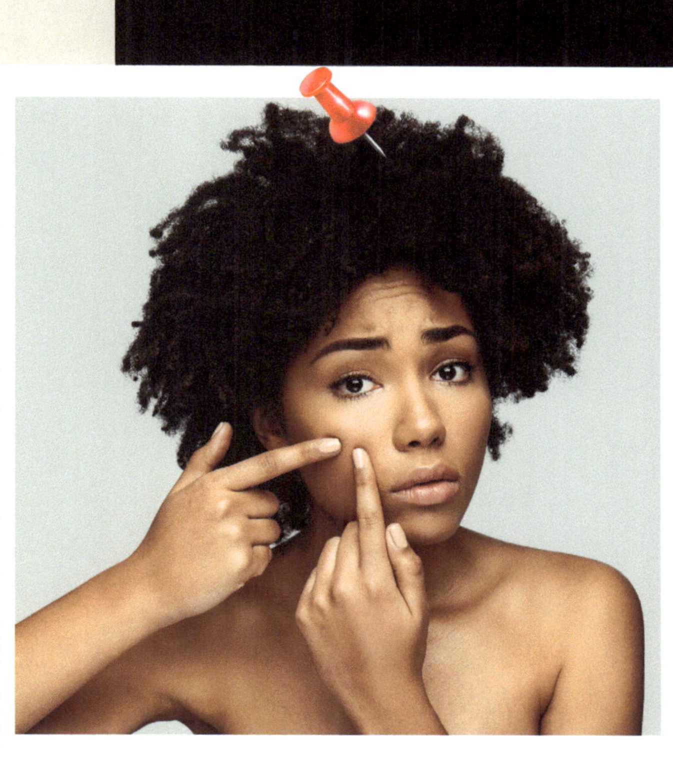

COMMON SKIN PROBLEMS

Psoriasis
Psoriasis is an autoimmune skin condition that causes the rapid buildup of skin cells, leading to thick, red, and scaly patches. It is believed to be caused by genetics and an overactive immune system.

Rosacea
Rosacea is a chronic skin condition characterized by facial redness, flushing, visible blood vessels, and sometimes pimples and swelling. It is more common in fair-skinned individuals and may be triggered by certain foods, alcohol, stress, and sun exposure.

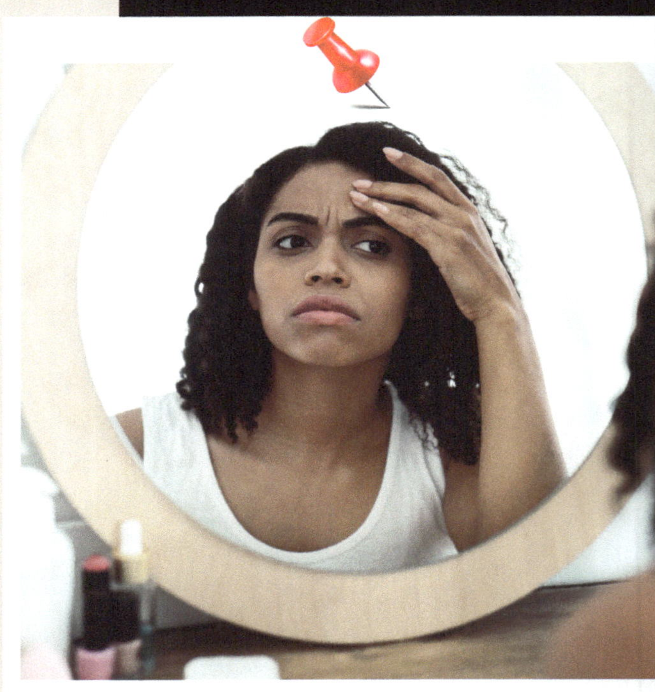

Hyperpigmentation
Hyperpigmentation refers to darkening of certain areas of the skin caused by an excess production of melanin. It can be caused by various factors, including sun exposure, hormonal changes, and skin injuries.

COMMON SKIN PROBLEMS

Fine Lines and Wrinkles

Fine lines and wrinkles are a natural part of the aging process. They are caused by a combination of factors, including sun exposure, collagen and elastin breakdown, and repetitive facial movements.

Dry Skin

Dry skin is characterized by a lack of moisture and can feel tight, itchy, and rough. It can be caused by genetic factors, environmental factors, and certain medications.

Oily Skin

Oily skin is characterized by excessive oil production, leading to a shiny complexion and a higher risk of developing acne. It is caused by genetic factors and hormonal changes.

Sensitive Skin

Sensitive skin is easily irritated and prone to redness, itching, and inflammation. It can be caused by genetic factors, environmental factors, and certain skincare products.

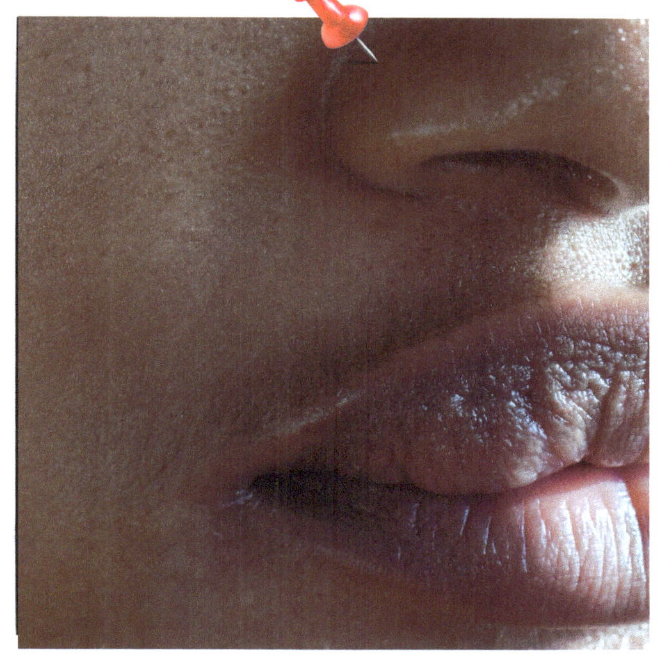

MY SKIN PROBLEM(S)

Note your skin problems as they outline the basis for your skincare goals. You will also need to be specific as this helps when selecting products for your skincare routine.

____

____

____

____

____

____

____

____

____

____

____

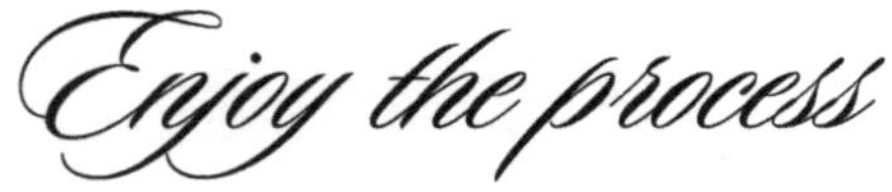

"GLOWING SKIN IS A result OF PROPER skincare."

CHAPTER

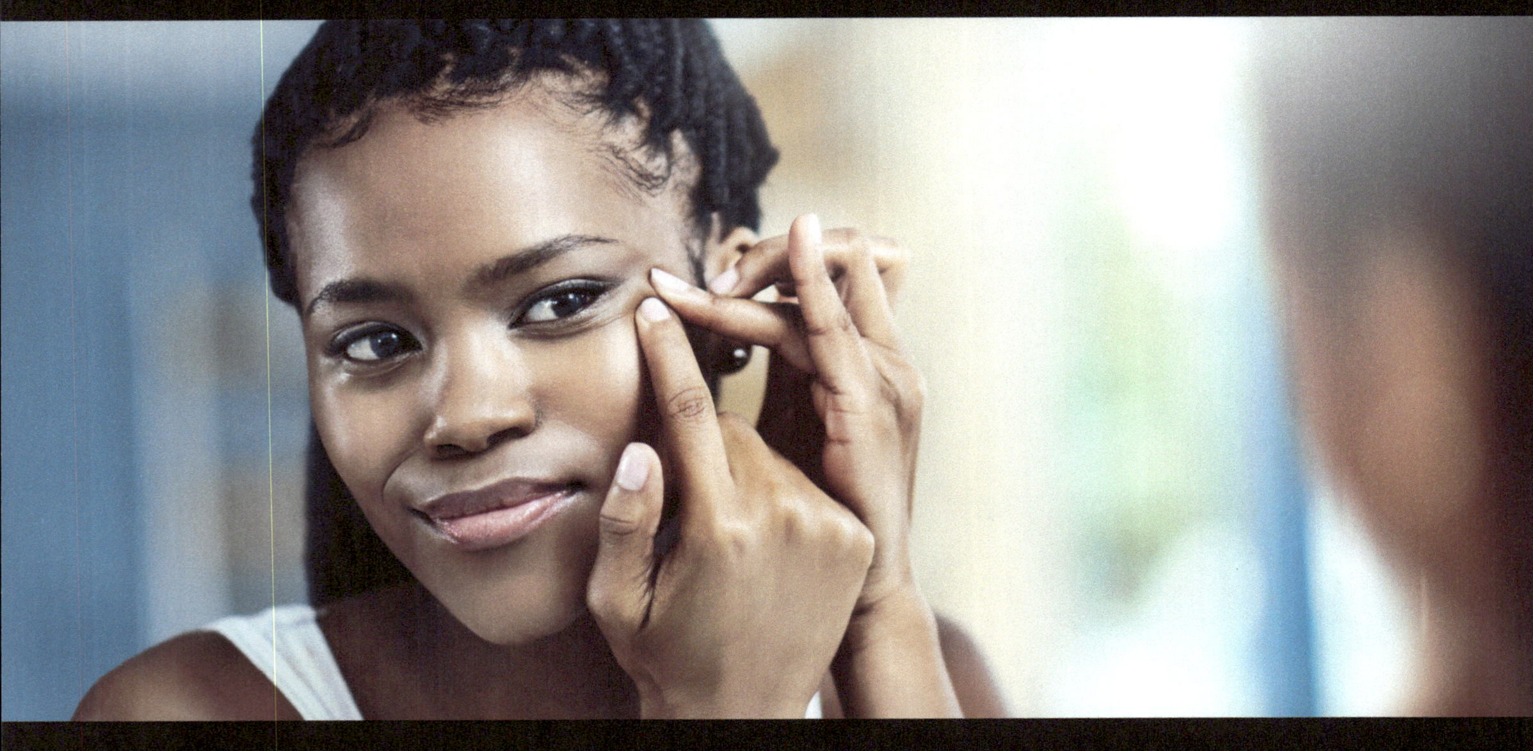

3

CAUSES OF SKIN PROBLEMS

1 PAGE

LET'S DO IT

SOPHIA BOWES

WORKBOOK

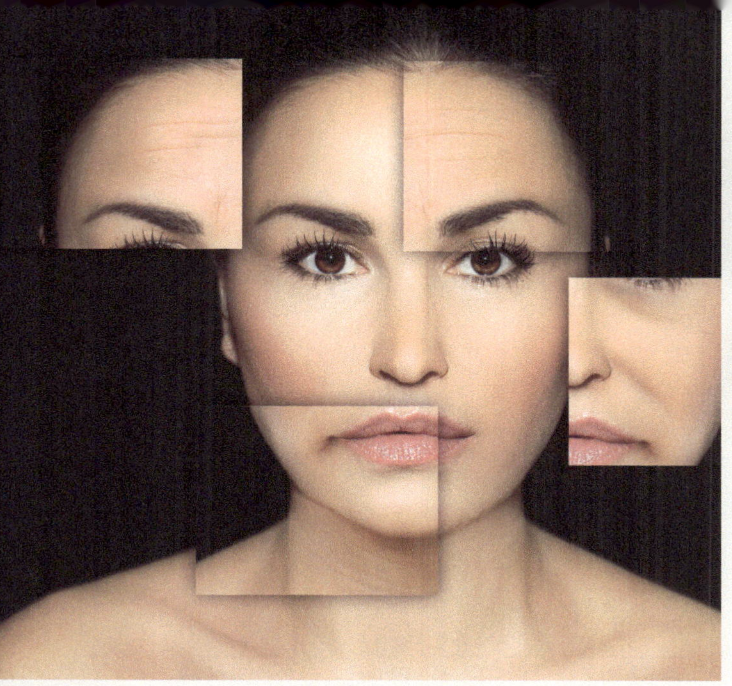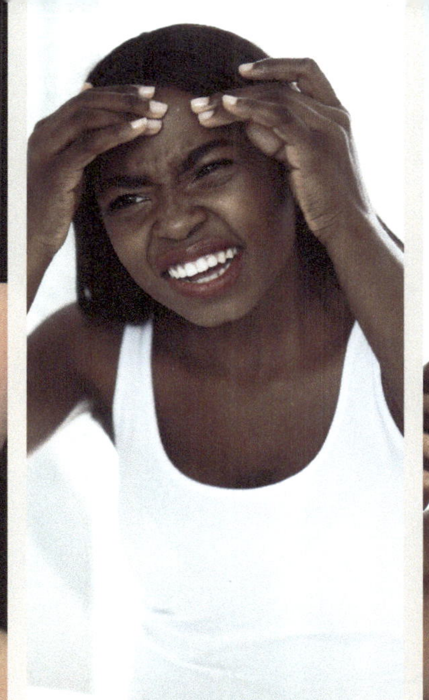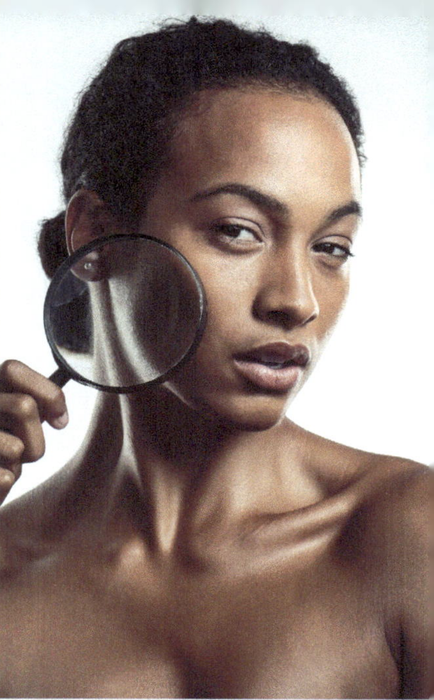

CAUSES OF SKIN PROBLEMS

Understanding the underlying causes of skin problems can help you address them more effectively. In this section, we will explore the various factors that contribute to the development of common skin problems.

Hormonal Imbalances

Hormonal imbalances, such as those that occur during puberty, menstruation, pregnancy, and menopause, can contribute to the development of acne and other skin problems.

Genetics

Genetic factors play a significant role in determining your skin type and susceptibility to certain skin conditions. If your parents have a history of acne, eczema, or other skin problems, you may be more likely to develop them as well.

Environmental Factors

Exposure to environmental factors, such as pollution, harsh weather conditions, and UV radiation, can damage the skin and contribute to the development of various skin problems.

Diet and Lifestyle

Poor diet and unhealthy lifestyle choices, such as smoking, excessive alcohol consumption, and lack of sleep, can negatively impact your skin's health and contribute to the development of skin problems.

Stress

Chronic stress can disrupt the balance of hormones in your body, leading to the development or exacerbation of skin problems, such as acne and eczema.

Incorrect Skincare Products/Routine

Using the wrong skincare products or following an incorrect skincare routine can disrupt your skin's natural balance and contribute to the development of skin problems.

CAUSE OF MY SKIN PROBLEM(S)

It is very important to identify the cause of your skincare problems because it gives you the best insight to treating, achieving and maintaining the desired results .

____

____

____

____

____

____

____

____

____

____

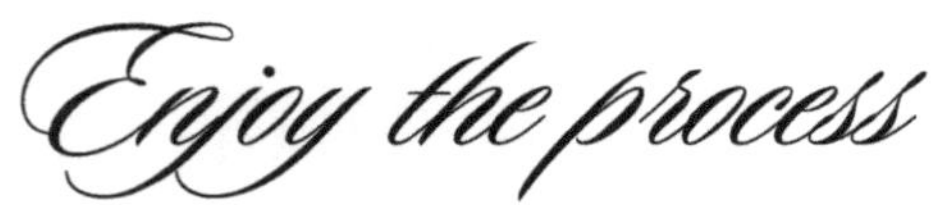

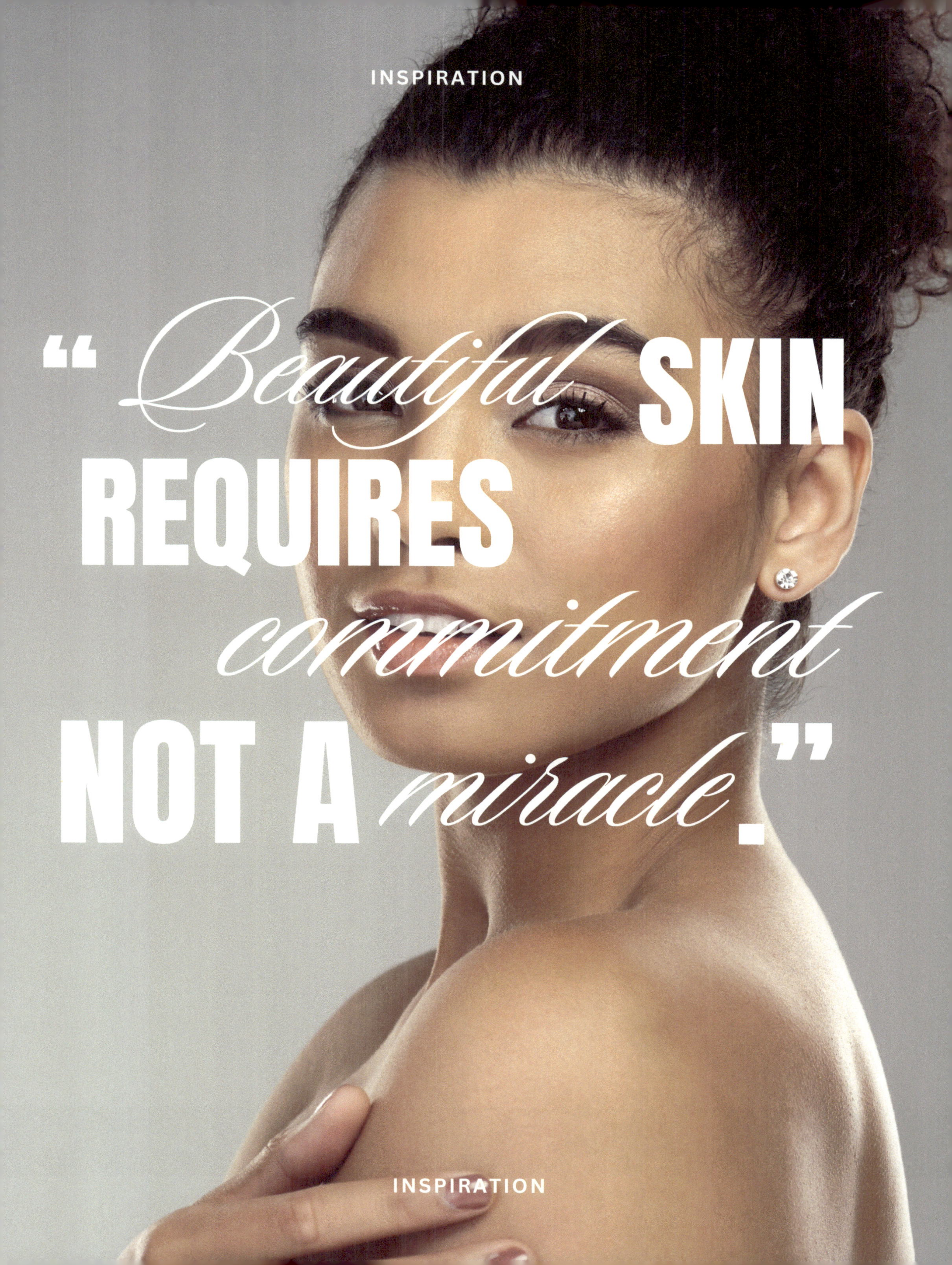

"*Beautiful* SKIN REQUIRES *commitment* NOT A *miracle*."

CHAPTER

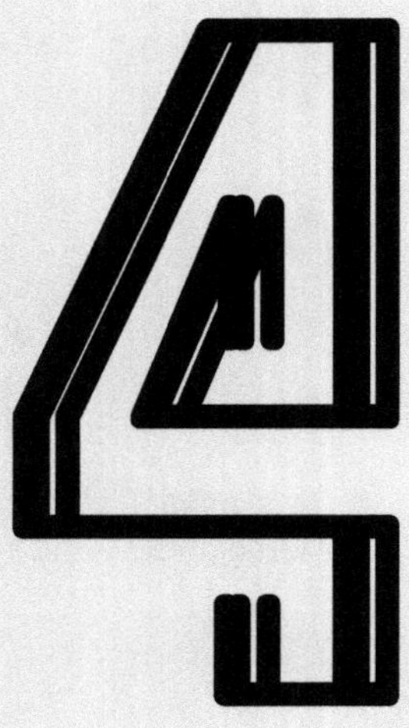

EFFECTIVE SOLUTIONS FOR RADIANT SKIN

2 PAGES

LET'S DO IT

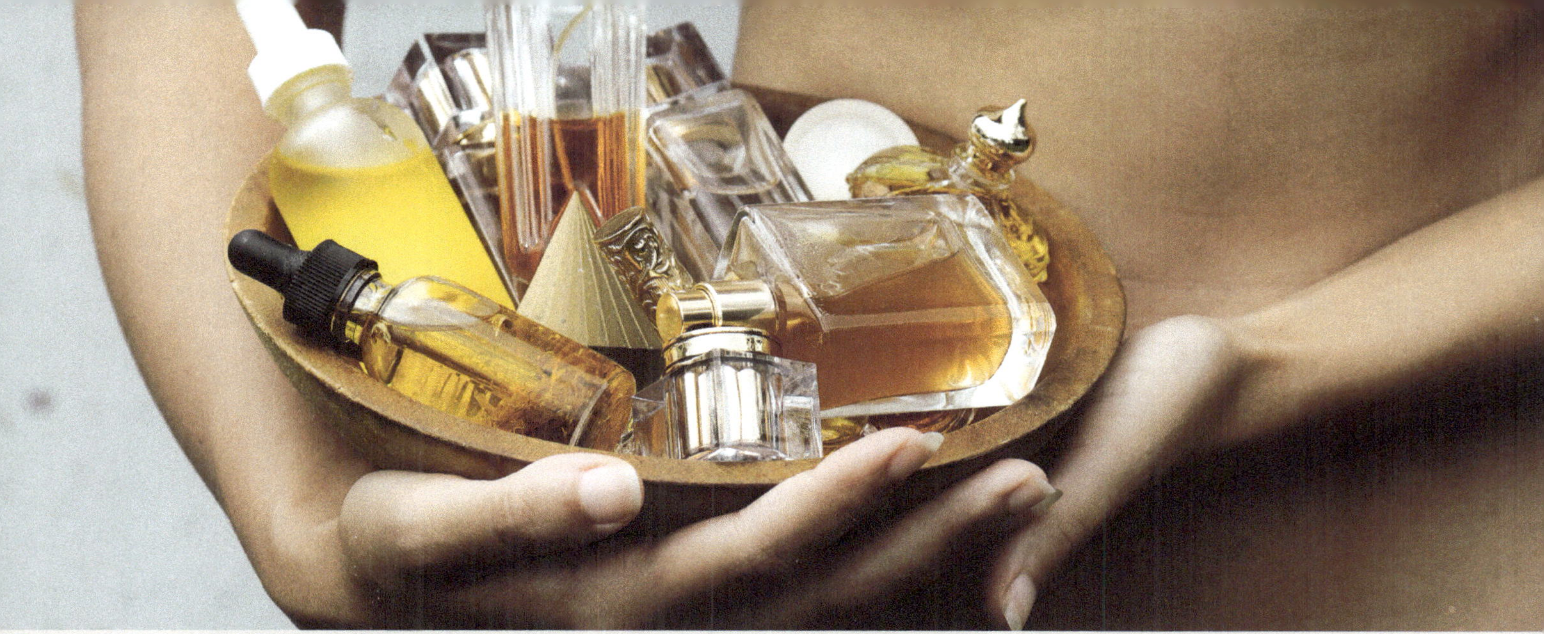

EFFECTIVE SOLUTIONS FOR RADIANT SKIN

Achieving clear and radiant skin requires a combination of healthy lifestyle habits, a consistent skincare routine, and the use of effective skincare products. In this section, we will explore various solutions that can help you achieve your skincare goals.

Protect from the Sun

Sun protection is crucial to prevent skin damage, premature aging, and the development of skin cancer. Use a broad-spectrum sunscreen with an SPF of 30 or higher daily, even on cloudy days.

Cleanse and Exfoliate

Cleansing your skin twice a day with a gentle cleanser helps remove dirt, oil, and impurities, preventing clogged pores and breakouts, view our range of natural cleansers here.

Exfoliating once or twice a week helps remove dead skin cells and promotes cell turnover, revealing a fresh and glowing complexion. We have a scrub that is just right for you.

Nutrition and Hydration

A balanced diet rich in fruits, vegetables, whole grains, and lean proteins provides essential nutrients for healthy skin. Additionally, staying hydrated by drinking an adequate amount of water helps maintain skin elasticity and overall health.

EFFECTIVE SOLUTIONS FOR RADIANT SKIN

Moisturize
Regardless of your skin type, moisturizing is essential to maintain hydrated and healthy skin. Choose a moisturizer that suits your skin type and contains ingredients like hyaluronic acid and ceramides to lock in moisture. Find moisture locking serums and moisturisers.

Manage Stress
Implement stress management techniques such as meditation, deep breathing exercises, and regular physical activity to reduce stress levels. High-stress levels can contribute to skin problems and accelerate the aging process.

Avoid Harsh Chemicals
Avoid skincare products that contain harsh chemicals, fragrances, and alcohol, as they can irritate the skin and exacerbate existing skin problems. Opt for gentle and natural skincare products instead.

Seek Professional Help
If you're struggling with persistent skin problems or are unsure about the best course of action, consult a dermatologist. They can provide personalized advice, prescribe medications if necessary, and recommend professional treatments.

CHAPTER

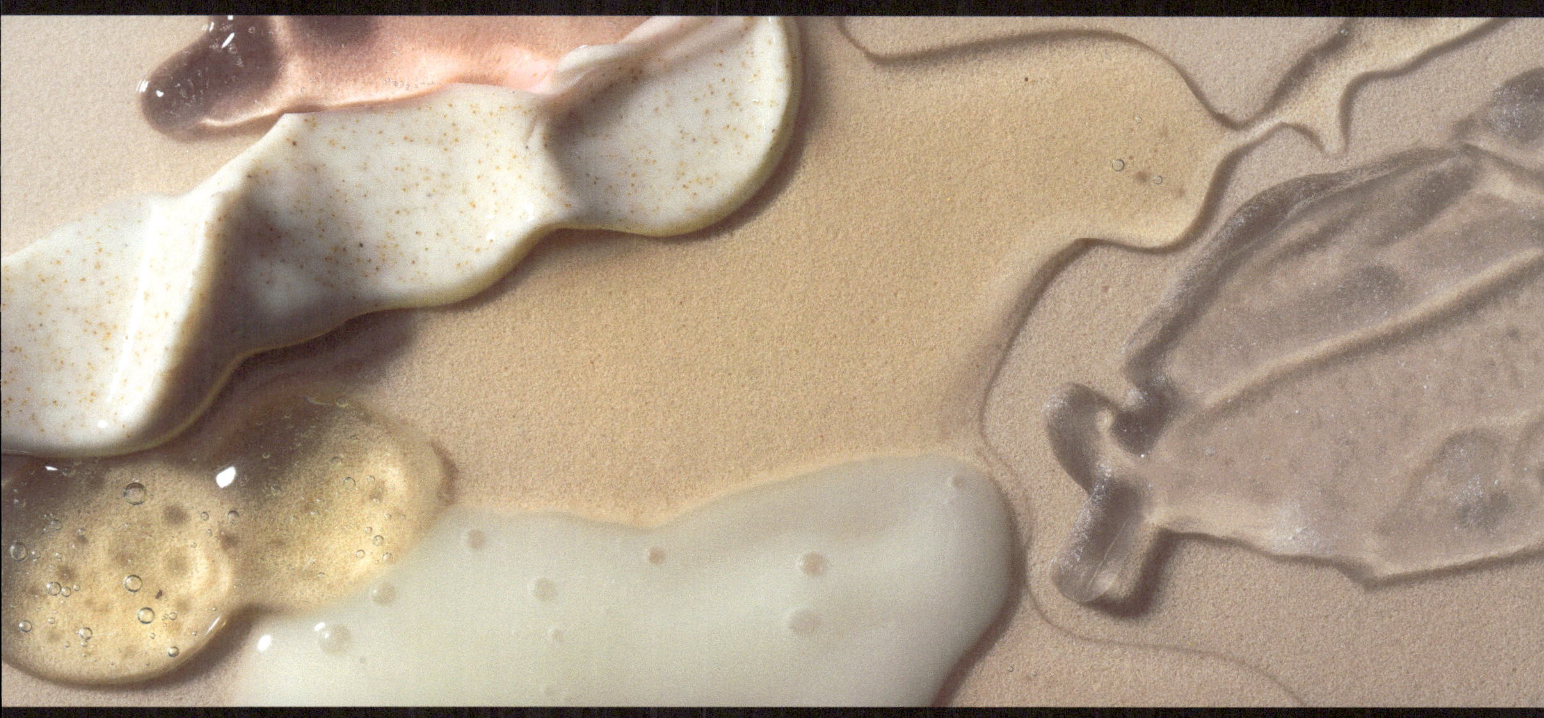

5

SKINCARE INGREDIENTS TO LOOK FOR

1 PAGE

LET'S
DO IT

SKINCARE INGREDIENTS TO LOOK FOR

Certain skincare ingredients have proven benefits for various skin concerns. Incorporating products that contain these ingredients into your skincare routine can help address specific skin problems effectively.

Retinoids

Retinoids, such as retinol and tretinoin, are vitamin A derivatives that promote cell turnover, reduce the appearance of fine lines and wrinkles, and improve overall skin texture. Skin Recovery Cream

Vitamin C

Vitamin C is a potent antioxidant that brightens the skin, reduces hyperpigmentation, and stimulates collagen production. Look for stable forms of vitamin C, such as L-ascorbic acid, in your skincare products.

Hyaluronic Acid

Hyaluronic acid is a humectant that attracts and retains moisture in the skin, keeping it hydrated and plump It helps reduce the appearance of fine lines and wrinkles and improves overall skin texture. Hyaluronic Acid Serum

Niacinamide

Niacinamide, also known as vitamin B3, helps regulate oil production, minimizes pore size, and reduces the appearance of hyperpigmentation and redness. Niacinamide Serum

Antioxidants

Antioxidants, such as vitamin E and green tea extract, help protect the skin from free radical damage, promote collagen production, and improve overall skin health.

CHOOSE MY INGREDIENTS/PRODUCTS

Select ingredients from our list based on skin type and problems you identified earlier in chapters 1 and 2.

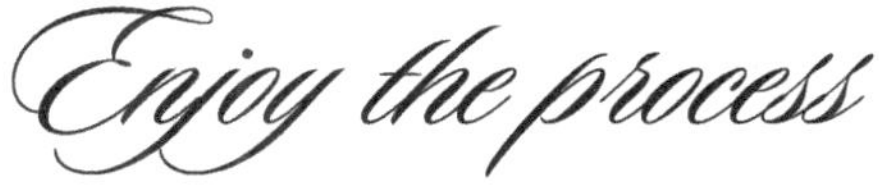

STAY FOCUSEDON YOUR OWN *unique* JOURNEY AND CELEBRATE YOUR *progress.*

CHAPTER

6

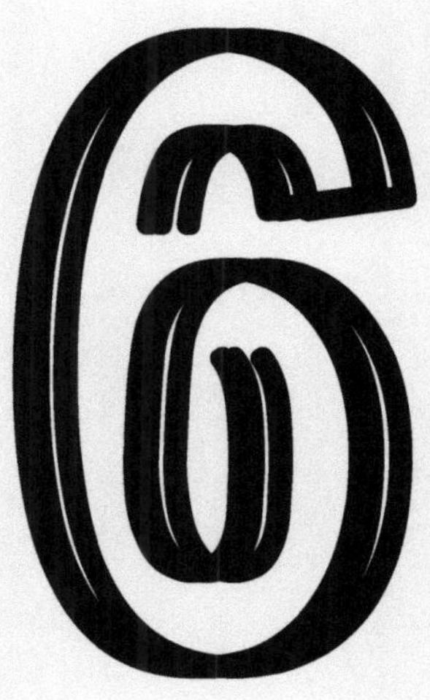

DAILY SKINCARE ROUTINE FOR CLEAR RADIANT SKIN

10 PAGES

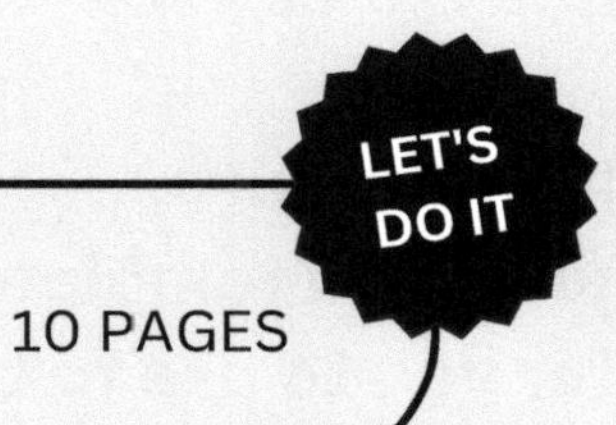

DAILY SKINCARE ROUTINE FOR CLEAR RADIANT SKIN

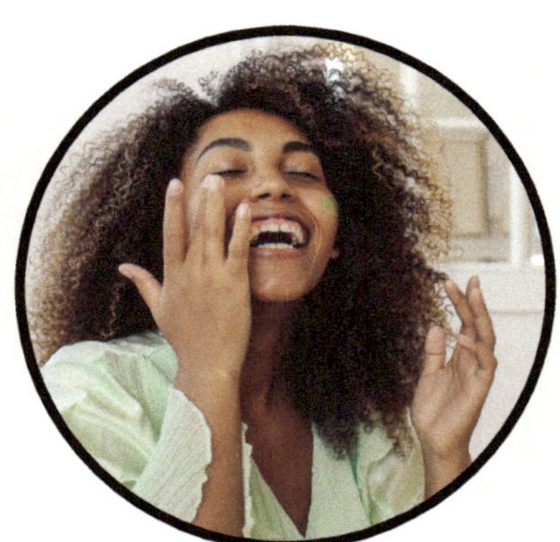

Establishing a consistent daily skincare routine is crucial for maintaining clear and radiant skin. In this section, we outline a basic skincare routine that can be tailored to your specific skin type and concerns.

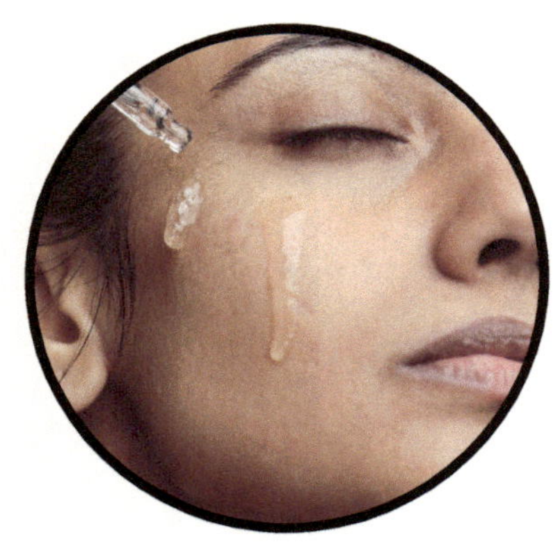

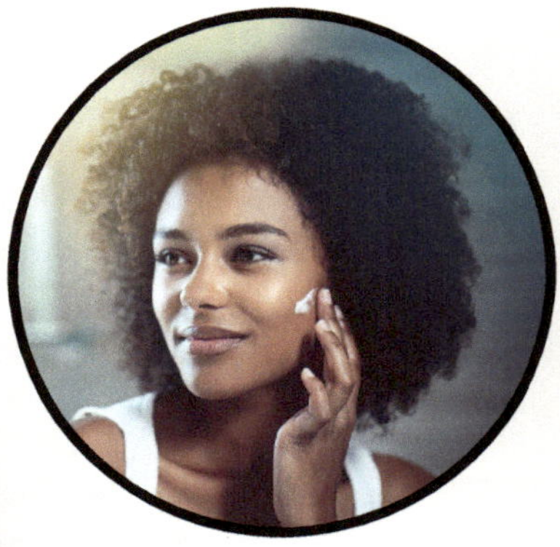

We have also, provided templates for you to use to build your own skincare routine while relying on the information from previous chapters as a guide.

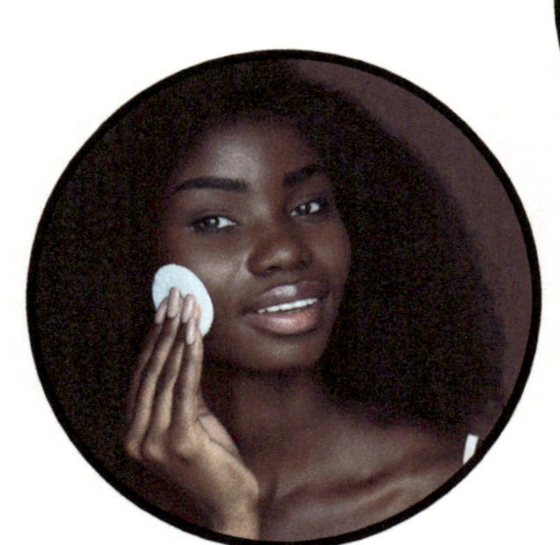

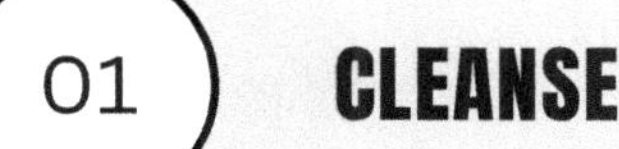

Basic Morning
SKINCARE ROUTINE

01

CLEANSE

Cleanse your face with a gentle cleanser to remove any impurities accumulated overnight.

02

TONE

Apply a toner to balance the skin's pH levels and prepare it for subsequent skincare products.

03

TREAT

Apply a serum or treatment product targeting your specific skin concerns, such as acne, hyperpigmentation, or aging.

04

MOISTURIZE

Moisturize your skin with a lightweight moisturizer suitable for your skin type.

05

PROTECT

Apply a broad-spectrum sunscreen with an SPF of 30 or higher, making sure to cover all exposed areas.

Basic Evening SKINCARE ROUTINE

01

CLEANSE

Remove makeup and cleanse your face thoroughly to remove any dirt, oil, and impurities accumulated throughout the day.

02

TONE - BALANCING

Use a toner to rebalance the skin's pH levels and remove any remaining traces of cleanser.

03

TREAT

Apply a serum or treatment product targeting your specific skin concerns.

04

MOISTURIZE

Moisturize your skin with a richer moisturizer to provide hydration and support the skin's natural repair process during sleep.

05

APPLY EYE TREATMENT

Apply an eye cream to target the delicate skin around the eyes.

06

EXFOLIATE

Incorporate a weekly exfoliation treatment to remove dead skin cells and promote cell turnover. You can start with 2 times per week.

Sample

DAILY SKINCARE *Routine*

Date:

Morning

1. **Cleanser:** Koji Brite Soap
2. **Toner:** Witch Hazel Toner
3. **Serum:** Niacinamide Serum
4. **Moisturizer:** Hyaluronic Acid Serum
5. **Sunscreen:** Your choice

Products to buy

- [ ]
- [ ]
- [ ]
- [ ]
- [ ]
- [ ]
- [ ]

Evening

1. **Remover:** Witch Hazel/ Your choice
2. **Face Scrub:** Turmeric Lemon Scrub
3. **Cleanser:** Koji Brite Soap
4. **Toner:** Honey Glow Elixir
5. **Serum:** Koji Brite Serum
6. **Moisturizer:** Skin Recovery Cream
7. **Eye Cream:** Your choice
8. **AHA/BHA:** Salicylic Acid optional
9. **Night Cream:** Your choice optional
10. **Mask:** Pink Clay Masque

Notes

Routine for spots and hyperpigmentation for oily skin type

Skincare Weekly Routine

Sample

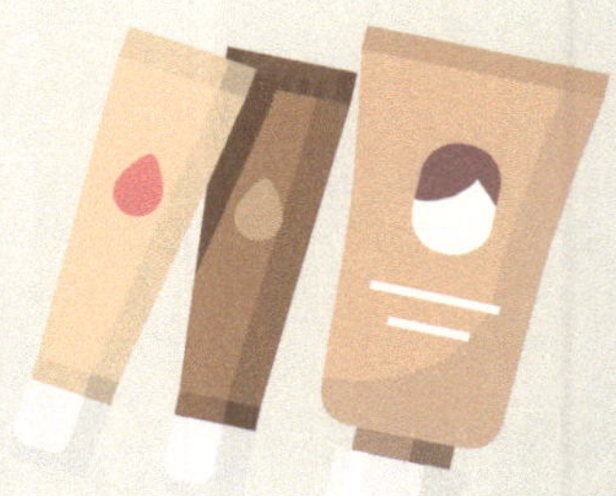

Monday

AM standard routine
Cleanse, tone, treat, moisturize, apply sunscreen

PM routine 1 through 7 & 9
Remove makeup, exfoliate, cleanse, tone, treat, moisturize, apply eye cream & night cream

Tuesday

AM standard routine
Cleanse, tone, treat, moisturize, apply sunscreen

PM routine 1, 3, 4, 8, 6, 7 & 9
Remove makeup, cleanse, tone, treat, moisturize, apply eye cream & night cream

Wednesday

AM standard routine
Cleanse, tone, treat, moisturize, apply sunscreen

PM routine 1, 10, 3 - 7 & 9
Remove makeup, cleanse, apply mask, tone, treat, moisturize, apply eye cream & night cream

Thursday

AM standard routine
Cleanse, tone, treat, moisturize, apply sunscreen

PM routine 1, 3, 4, 8, 6 , 7 & 9
Remove makeup, cleanse, tone, treat, moisturize, apply eye cream & night cream

Friday

AM standard routine
Cleanse, tone, treat, moisturize, apply sunscreen

PM routine 1 through 7 & 9
Remove makeup, exfoliate, cleanse, tone, treat, moisturize, apply eye cream & night cream

Saturday

AM standard routine
Cleanse, tone, treat, moisturize, apply sunscreen

PM routine 1, 10, 3 - 7 & 9
Remove makeup, cleanse, apply mask, tone, treat, moisturize, apply eye cream & night cream

---

Notes :
Weekly skincare routine.
Apply products from light to heavy and allow 1 or 2 minutes between applications.
Drink 8 glasses of water daily.

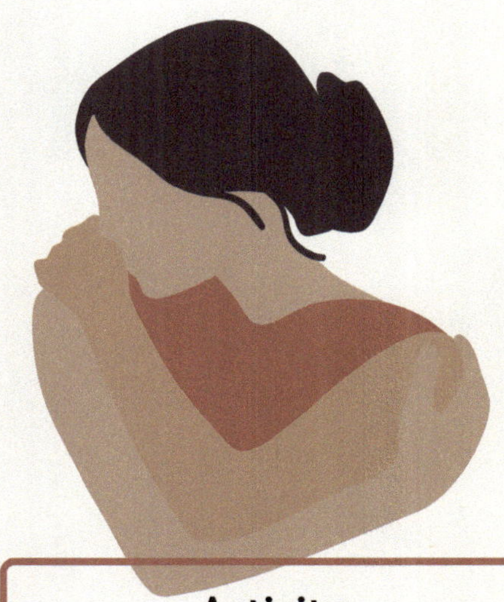

SAMPLE
DAILY ROUTINE TRACKER

Date:

Activity	S	M	T	W	T	F	S
Wake up							
Shower							
Morning Skin Routine							
Eat Breakfast							
Work/ Days activity							
Exercise							
Shower							
Dinner							
Prepare for next day							
Evening Skin Routine							
Bed							

Build My Morning
SKINCARE ROUTINE

Visit our website <u>here</u> and select products for the different categories below to add to your skincare routine builder. Or use your current products.

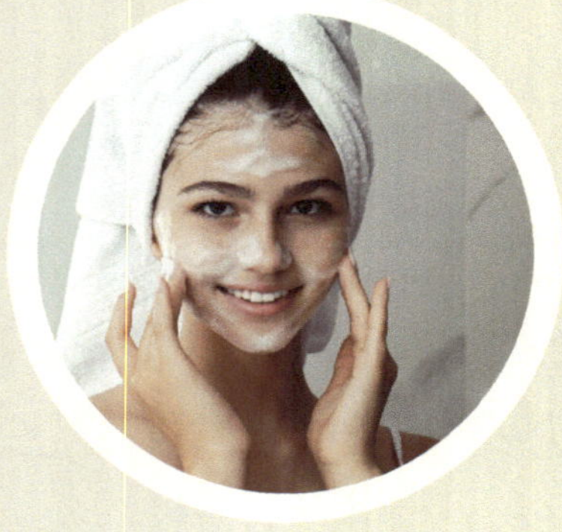

CLEANSER - SOAP OR FOAM WASH

____

____

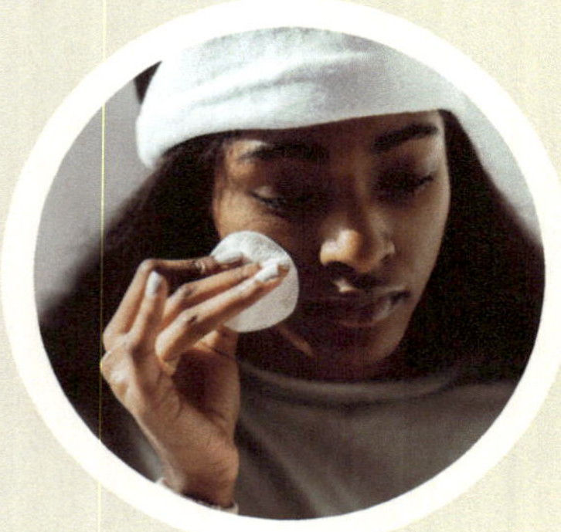

TONER

____

____

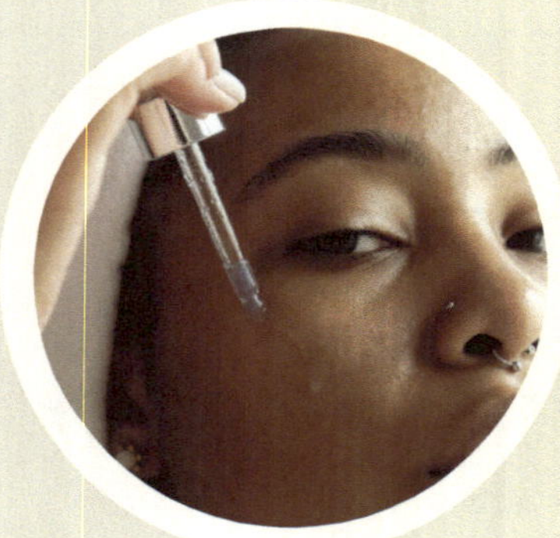

SERUM

____

____

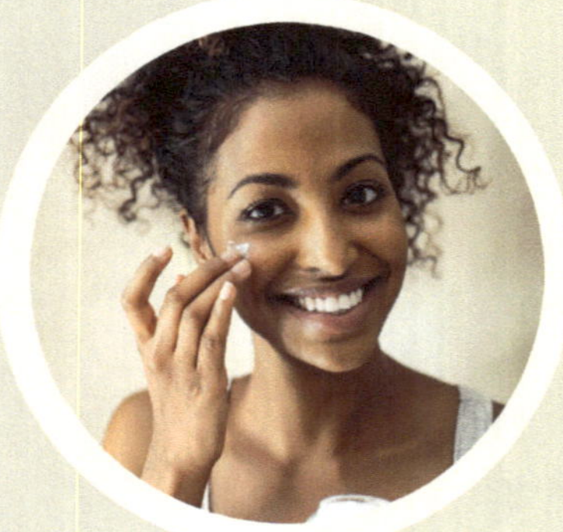

MOISTURISER

____

____

Ensure products added here are specific to your skin type and problem.

Build My Evening
SKINCARE ROUTINE

Visit our website <u>here</u> and select products for the different categories below to add to your skincare routine builder. Or use your current products.

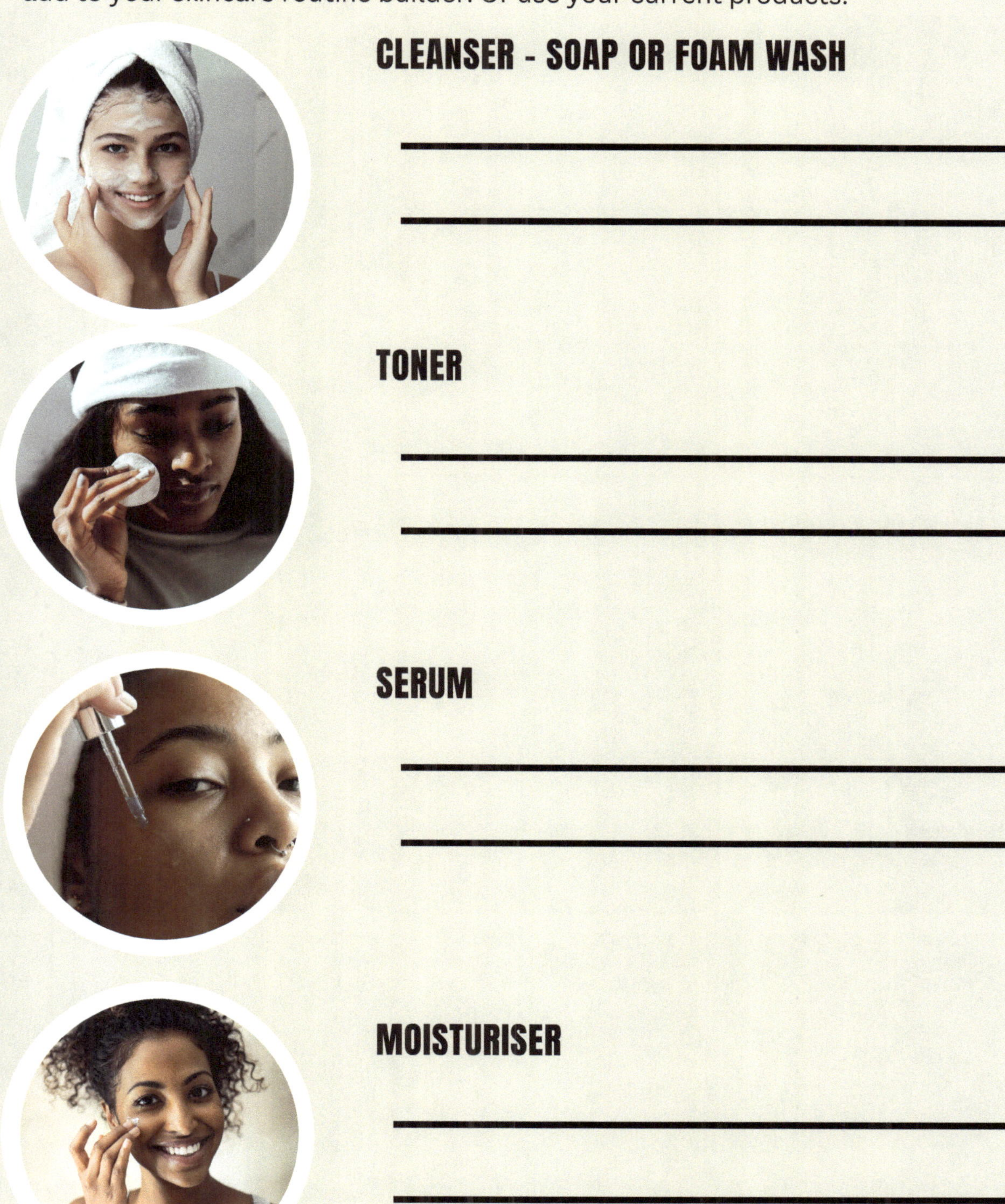

CLEANSER - SOAP OR FOAM WASH

____

____

TONER

____

____

SERUM

____

____

MOISTURISER

____

____

Ensure products added here are specific to your skin type and problem.

My **Skincare Weekly Routine**

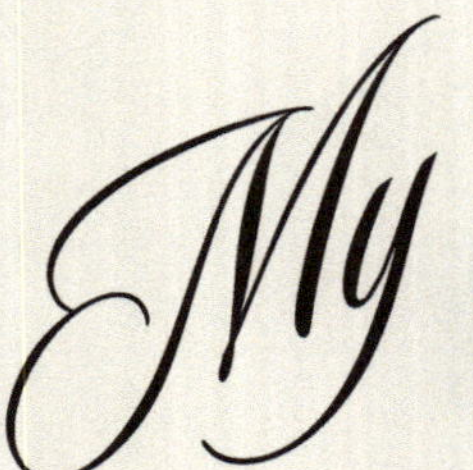

Monday

Tuesday

Wednesday

Thursday

Friday

Saturday

Notes :
Weekly skincare routine.
Apply products from light to heavy and allow 1 or 2 minutes
between applications.
Drink 8 glasses of water daily.

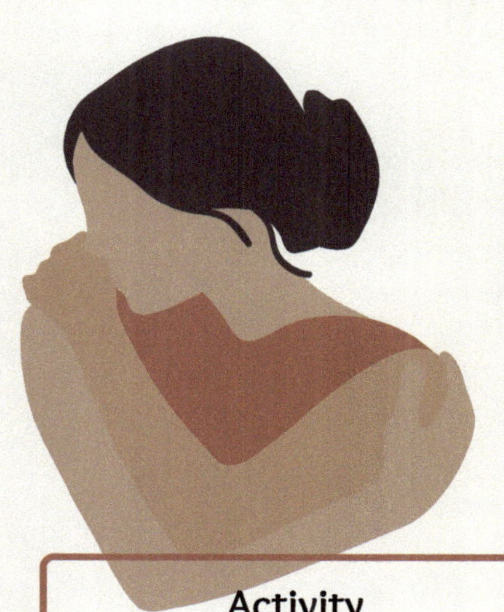

MY DAILY ROUTINE TRACKER

Date:

Activity	S	M	T	W	T	F	S

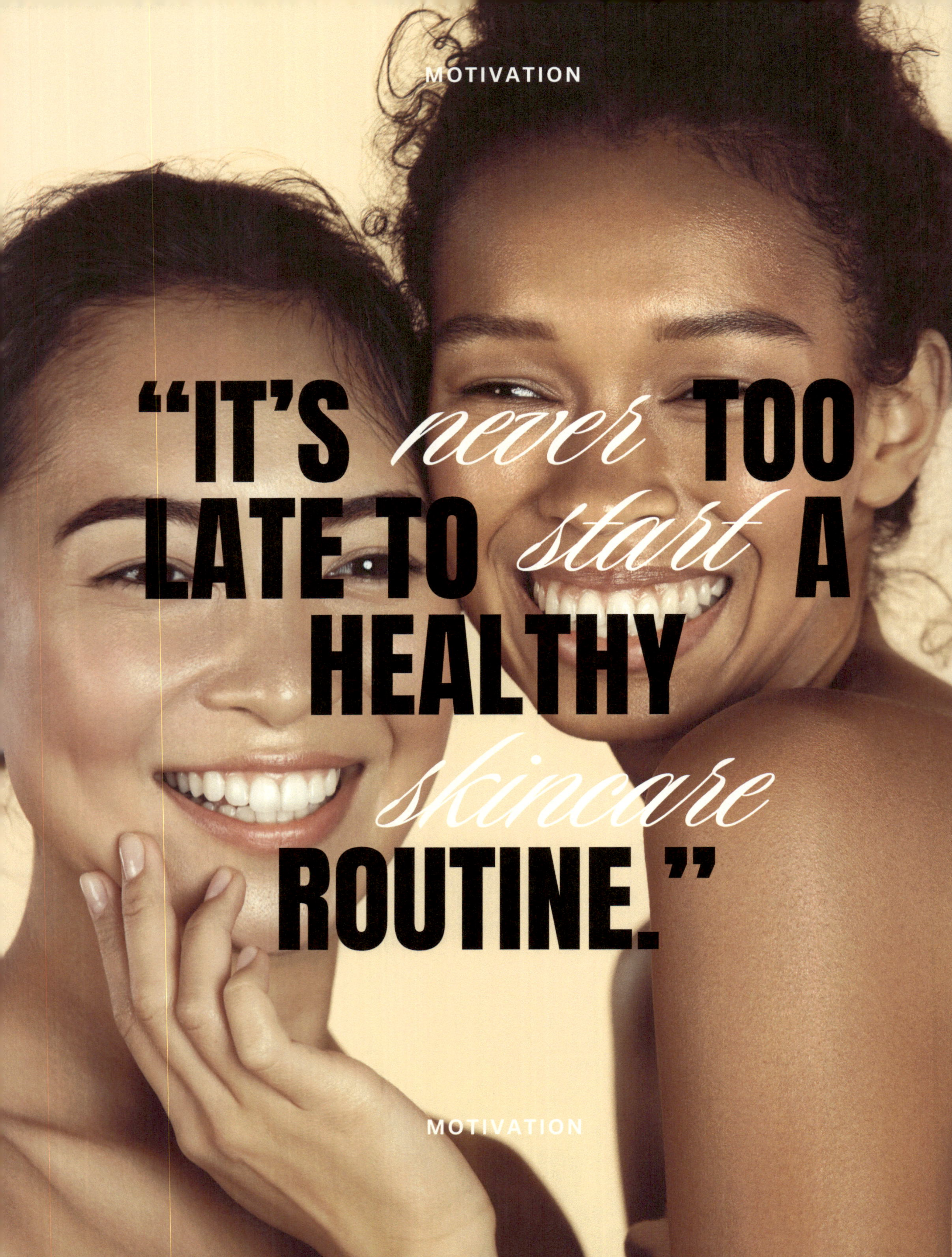
"IT'S never TOO LATE TO start A HEALTHY skincare ROUTINE."

CHAPTER

helpful tips

7

LIFESTYLE TIPS FOR HEALTHY SKIN

1 PAGE

LET'S DO IT

LIFESTYLE TIPS FOR HEALTHY SKIN

In addition to a consistent skincare routine, certain lifestyle habits can contribute to healthy, clear, and radiant skin. In this section, we will explore various lifestyle tips to support your skincare efforts.

Diet and Nutrition

Maintain a balanced diet rich in fruits, vegetables, whole grains, lean proteins, and healthy fats. Limit your intake of processed foods, sugary snacks, and beverages as they can contribute to skin problems.

Exercise

Regular exercise promotes healthy blood circulation, which nourishes the skin with essential nutrients and oxygen. Aim for at least 30 minutes of moderate-intensity exercise most days of the week.

Hydration

Drink an adequate amount of water daily to keep your body hydrated. Hydration is essential for maintaining skin elasticity and overall health.

Sleep

Get enough quality sleep every night to allow your skin to repair and rejuvenate. Aim for 7-9 hours of uninterrupted sleep.

Stress Management

Practice stress management techniques, such as meditation, deep breathing exercises, and engaging in activities you enjoy. Chronic stress can contribute to skin problems, so it's essential to find healthy ways to manage stress.

Remember, gaining and maintaining healthy glowing skin is a holistic approach. You will not only look but feel better.

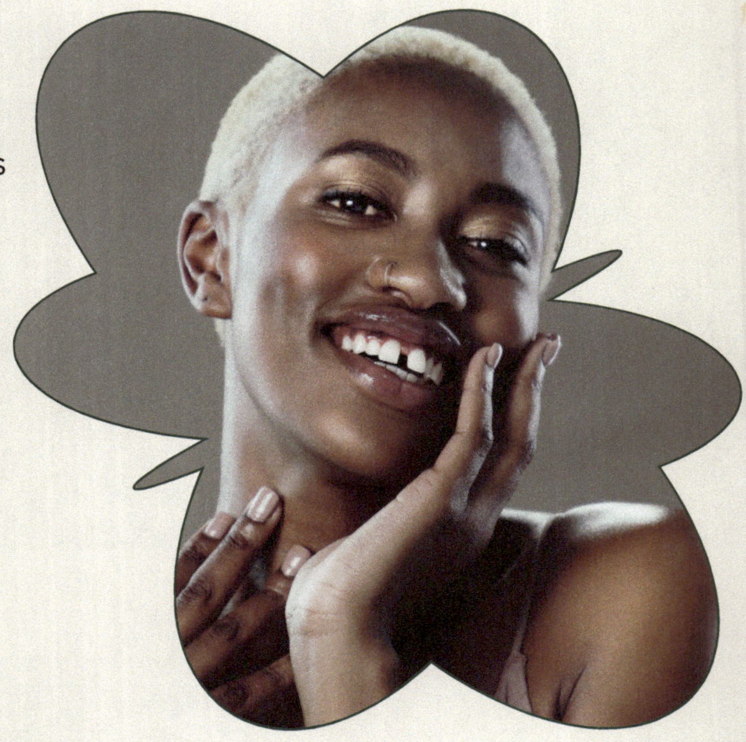

TIP(S) TO ADD TO MY ROUTINE

Identify the tips that you believe will enhance your routine if added.

Enjoy the process

STAY CONSISTENT
IN YOUR OWN
skincare JOURNEY
AND CELEBRATE
YOUR success.

CHAPTER

§

PROFESSIONAL TREATMENT FOR SKIN PROBLEMS

1 PAGE

LET'S DO IT

PROFESSIONAL TREATMENT FOR SKIN PROBLEMS

In some cases, professional treatments may be necessary to address specific skin problems. In this section, we will explore various professional treatments that can be effective in improving the appearance and health of your skin.

Chemical Peels
Chemical peels involve the application of a chemical solution to the skin to exfoliate the outermost layer. They can improve skin texture, reduce the appearance of fine lines and wrinkles, and even out skin tone.

Microdermabrasion
Microdermabrasion is a non-invasive procedure that uses a diamond-tipped wand or crystals to exfoliate the skin. It helps improve skin texture, reduce the appearance of fine lines and wrinkles, and stimulate collagen production.

Laser Therapy
Laser therapy uses focused beams of light to target specific skin concerns, such as acne scars, hyperpigmentation, and fine lines. It promotes collagen production and helps improve overall skin texture.

Dermabrasion
Dermabrasion involves the use of a rotating brush or diamond wheel to remove the outer layer of the skin. It is effective in treating scars, wrinkles, and sun-damaged skin.

Microneedling
Microneedling, also known as collagen induction therapy, uses tiny needles to create controlled micro-injuries in the skin. It stimulates collagen production and can improve the appearance of scars, wrinkles, and hyperpigmentation.

Remember, sometimes professional help may be needed especially if your skin issue is severe.

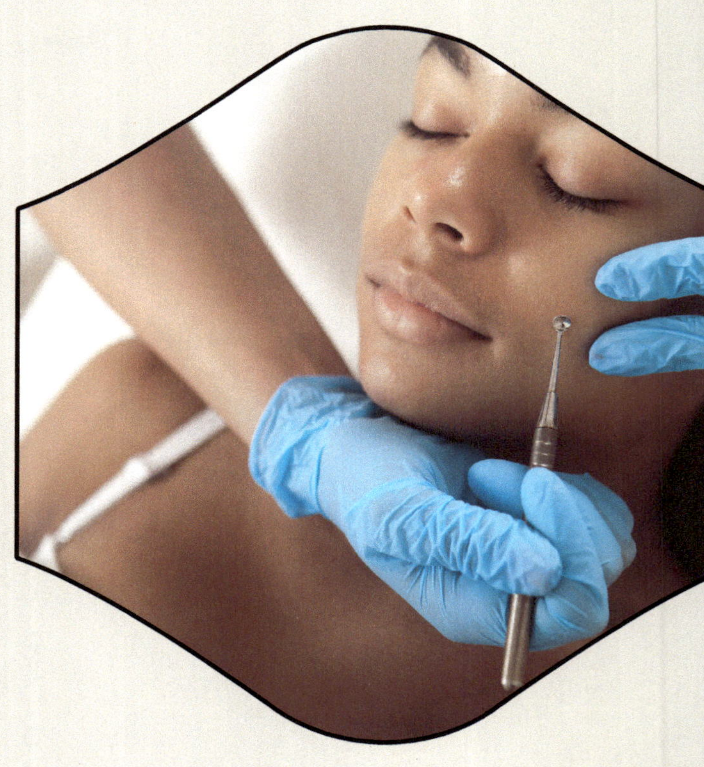

YOUR NOTES:

Enjoy the process

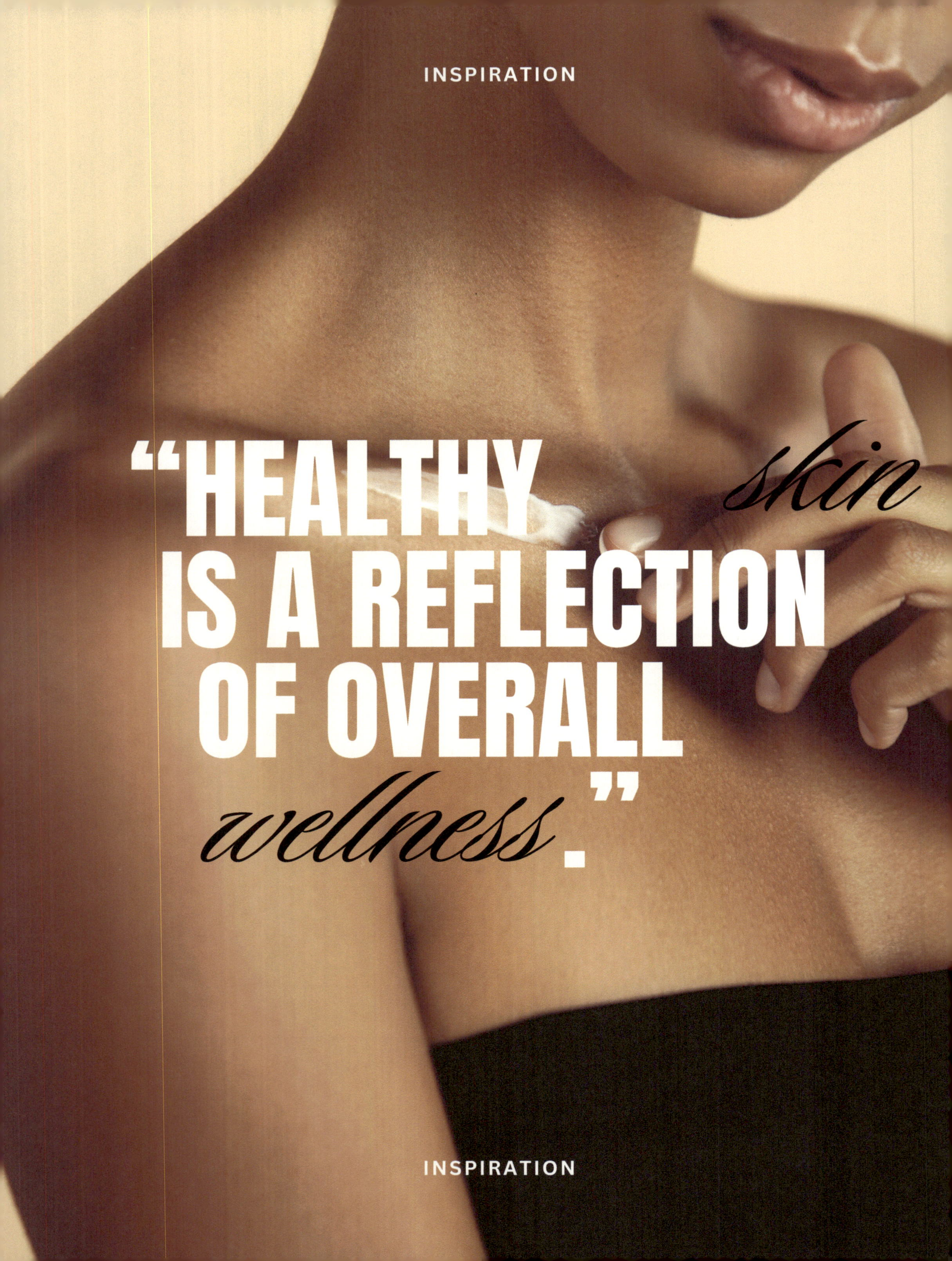

"HEALTHY *skin* IS A REFLECTION OF OVERALL *wellness*."

CHAPTER

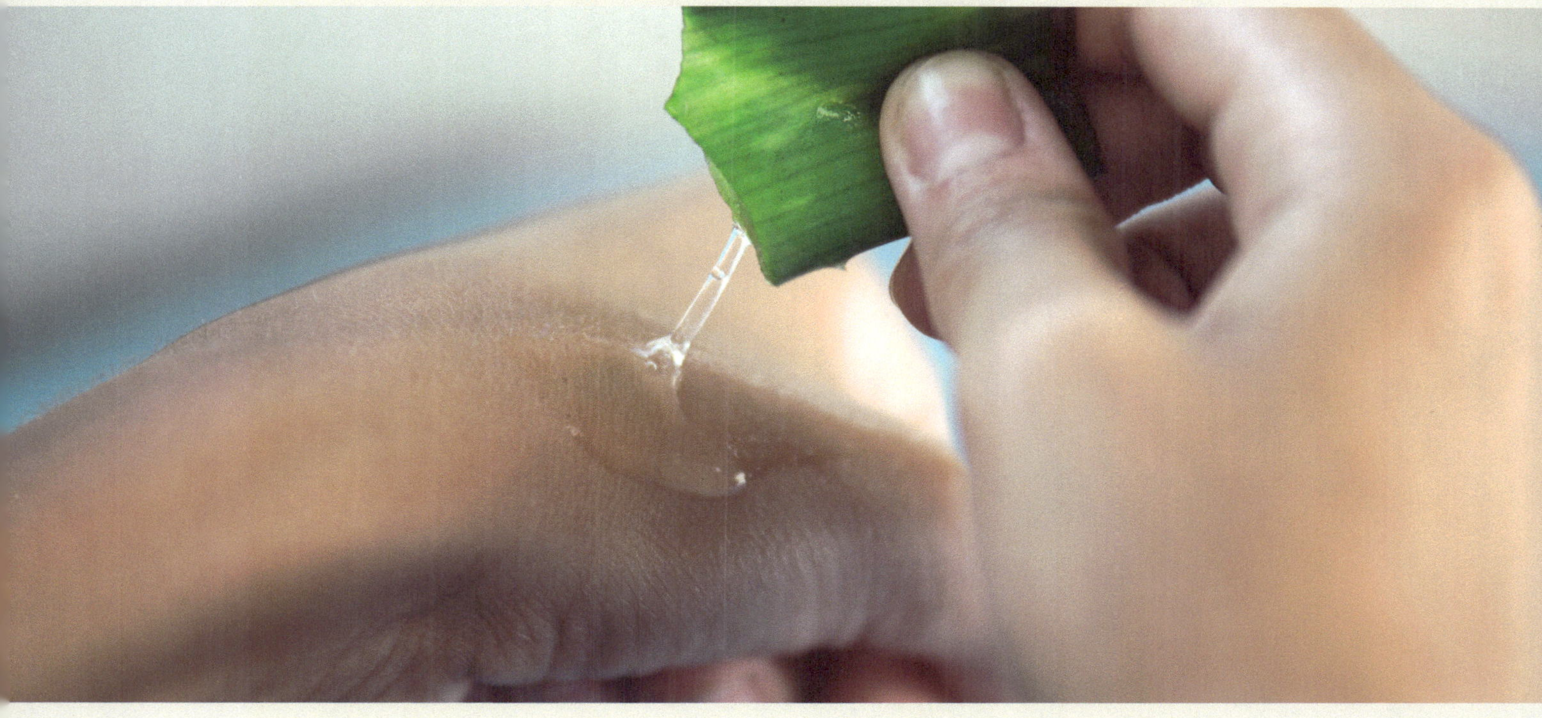

9

HOME REMEDIES FOR COMMON SKIN PROBLEMS

1 PAGE

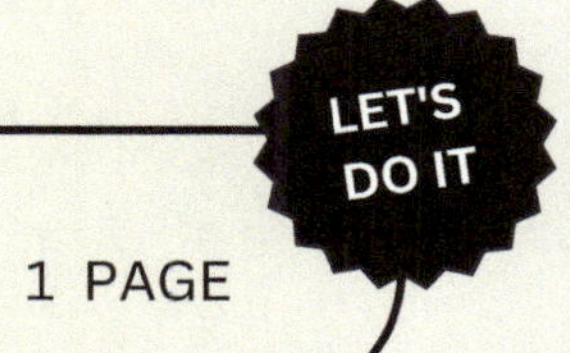

SOPHIA BOWES

WORKBOOK

HOME REMEDIES FOR COMMON SKIN PROBLEMS

In addition to professional treatments where necessary and a consistent skincare routine, certain home remedies can help address common skin problems. In this section, we will explore some effective home remedies for specific skin concerns.

Tea Tree Oil for Acne

Tea tree oil has antibacterial and anti-inflammatory properties that can help reduce acne breakouts. Dilute tea tree oil with a carrier oil and apply it to affected areas using a cotton swab.

Oatmeal Baths for Eczema

Taking oatmeal baths can soothe itchy and inflamed skin associated with eczema. Add colloidal oatmeal to warm bathwater and soak for 15-20 minutes.

Aloe Vera Gel for Sunburn

Aloe vera gel has cooling and soothing properties that can provide relief from sunburn. Apply aloe vera gel directly to sunburned areas for instant relief.

Apple Cider Vinegar for Hyperpigmentation

Apple cider vinegar can help lighten dark spots and hyperpigmentation. Mix equal parts apple cider vinegar and water, and apply the mixture to the affected areas using a cotton ball.

Rosehip Oil for Fine Lines and Wrinkles

Rosehip oil is rich in antioxidants and essential fatty acids that can improve the appearance of fine lines and wrinkles. Gently massage a few drops of rosehip oil onto clean skin before applying moisturizer.

CONCLUSION

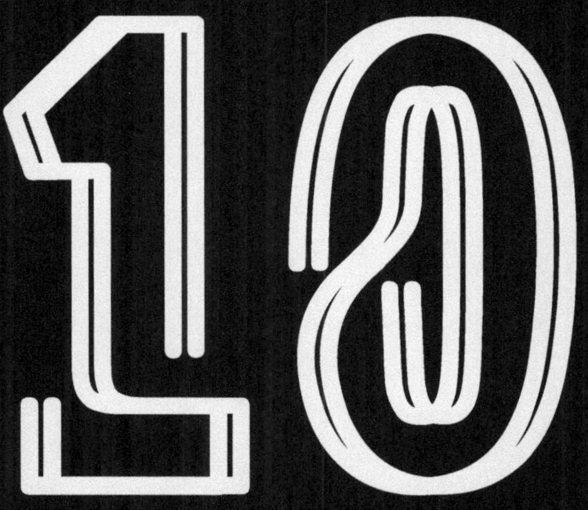

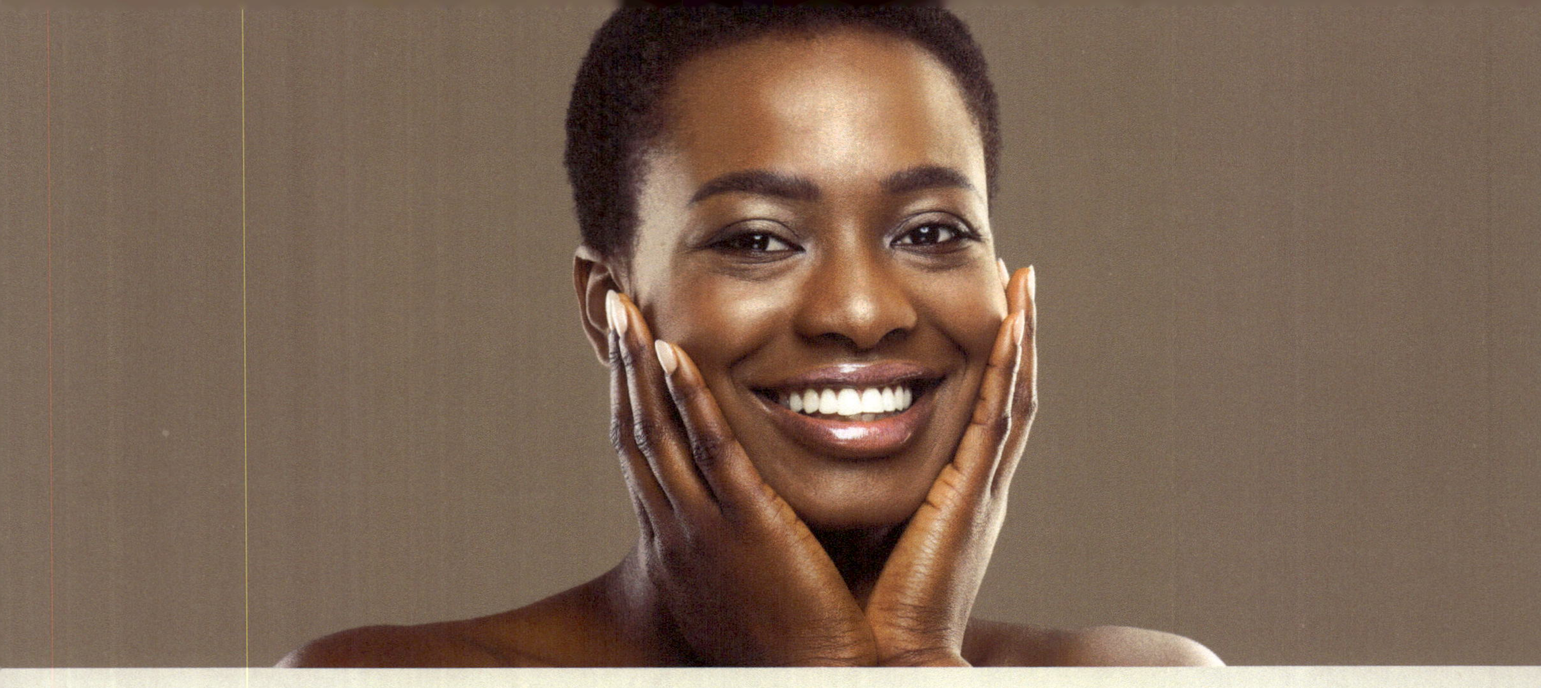

CONCLUSION

Achieving clear and radiant skin is possible with the right knowledge, skincare routine, and lifestyle habits. By understanding your skin type, identifying common skin problems, and implementing effective solutions, you can enhance the health and appearance of your skin. Remember to consult a dermatologist for personalized advice and professional treatments when necessary. With consistent care and a holistic approach, you can achieve the clear and radiant skin you desire.

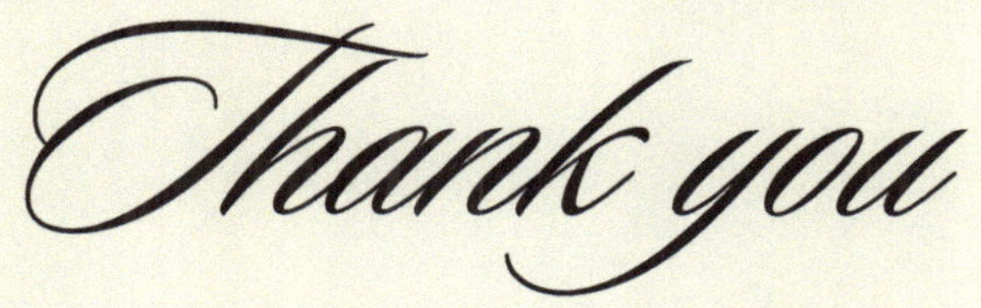

FOR READING

**CONGRATULATIONS ON COMPLETING THIS JOURNEY
TOWARDS ACHIEVING CLEAR RADIANT SKIN**

WWW.REJENSKINHAVEN.COM
@REJENSKINHAVEN

USE: EBOOK20 FOR
20% OFF $30